T0105574

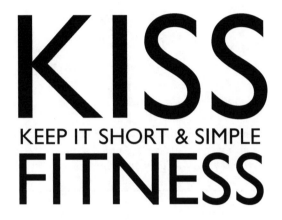

KISS
KEEP IT SHORT & SIMPLE
FITNESS

CAREY LONG

iUniverse, Inc.
New York   Bloomington

KISS FITNESS
Keep It Short & Simple

Copyright © 2010 by Carey Long
Cover Photography by Kevin C Davis
Interior Photography by Brian Baiamonte

All rights reserved. No part of this book may be used or reproduced by any means, graphic, electronic, or mechanical, including photocopying, recording, taping or by any information storage retrieval system without the written permission of the publisher except in the case of brief quotations embodied in critical articles and reviews.

iUniverse books may be ordered through booksellers or by contacting:
iUniverse
1663 Liberty Drive
Bloomington, IN 47403
www.iuniverse.com
1-800-Authors (1-800-288-4677)

Because of the dynamic nature of the Internet, any Web addresses or links contained in this book may have changed since publication and may no longer be valid. The views expressed in this work are solely those of the author and do not necessarily reflect the views of the publisher, and the publisher hereby disclaims any responsibility for them.

ISBN: 978-1-4502-2137-5 (pbk)
ISBN: 978-1-4502-2138-2 (ebk)

Printed in the United States of America

iUniverse rev. date: 9/1/10

Table of Contents

The KISS Fitness Approach

A practical plan for a longer life and a more attractive and healthier you

By Carey Long, Personal Trainer

Preface: A PERSONAL NOTE

HOW MUCH THOUGHT HAVE YOU GIVEN TO YOUR LIFE EXPECTANCY?

I never did until recently. Now that I have turned 40 this thought keeps creeping into my mind.

"But you're still young!" my friend exclaimed. "Don't waste your time worrying about something you can't change! When it's your time to go, you'll go. That's the way it is!"

"Really? You don't think there's anything I can do to change my life expectancy?" I responded to my friend.

Well, I thought about it and I do think there is something I can do to change my life expectancy! That is why I am writing this little book. It is for my friend and for the countless others who are holding onto a similar line of thinking.

Granted that none of us can ever be in total charge of our life expectancy, the unforeseen and unexpected happen. Both my parents died by 64 years of age; one of Lou Gehrig's disease and the other due to complications from multiple heart attacks. And probably just like you, I know people who have died in accidents.

I accept that these things do happen, but what I don't accept there is nothing I can do to increase the probability of having a longer life expectancy and equally important, a better quality of life for the years that I do live. I want to have a long life. I want to stay healthy. I want to be the most attractive me that I can be. Simply put, I want more time to continue enjoying life.

I have been exercising for over 22 years, but only understanding and realizing the best way to get in shape and stay in shape for about 10 years. Working as a licensed Physical Therapist Assistant and Certified Personal Trainer has only prepped me for service as a provider of training. But, more importantly, my life experience has provided me with the practical knowledge and know-how to help others. Through trial and error in working with the many personalities, needs, and desires of hundreds of very different clients, I now have an understanding of what works and what does not work and I want to share my experience with you.

Exercise and fitness do not need to be complicated to be effective. In fact, the title KISS is an acronym most of us are familiar with that stands for Keep It Simple Stupid. Follow me through this little book as I reveal a practical and effective plan that can make a big difference in both your life expectancy and the quality of your life. I promise you the journey will be worth your time and most important of all, we will take a complicated subject and make it easy to understand. We will turn Keep It Simple Stupid into **KEEP IT SHORT & SIMPLE.**

Chapter 1: WHY I INVESTED TIME BRINGING THE KISS FITNESS APPROACH TO YOU

Why this book?

There is so much information out there now via search engines and countless magazines but most share one short coming, overload of information. Maybe it is to make the author or trainer stand out. What I have found throughout this process is ultimately it comes down to the individual doing the work. If it appears too complicated, then it is more likely that the reader will perceive the information is too advanced or out of personal reach with just a few flips of a page.

Why me?

As mentioned before, I have been exercising for just over 22 years now but really understanding what it takes to achieve different levels of fitness in the last decade. I was fortunate to learn about exercise in the beginning from very knowledgeable people that were comfortable sharing information about what had worked for them in the past. The only issue was that most of the information was directed towards the body building physique. Bodybuilding physiques are considered so 1980's. Let's face it; it takes countless hours in the gym alongside a meticulous diet to maintain those larger muscles. Plus, I did not want a look that took away from an athletic appearance. My goal then was the same as it is now. I want people to see me as an athlete first. I want to be able to jump, run, and throw, etc., like I did as a kid.

So, to better understand the body and how it works in regards to form and function I went to school and became licensed as a Physical Therapist Assistant followed shortly after with a certification through the NSCA (National Strength and Conditioning Association). What I gained after this entry level of new knowledge was how to fix my parts that hurt while at the same time continuing to develop my whole body. Instead of trying to look like everyone else in the gym, I found a body type and look that I wanted. I started teaching spin classes almost

10 years ago to ensure that my cardio was at the level I needed to reach my new body type and improve my heart and lung function. This was a way for me to get in front of more individuals that wanted to increase their chance of living longer, healthier lives.

Over the course of the last 15 years until taking pictures for this book my bodyweight has changed a remarkable 40 plus pounds. Part of it was an effort to change my physique so that I could attract more clients, but another major factor was addressing my genetically driven health concerns. I still get questioned regularly about changing my workout approach to get bigger again and I simply do not want to carry around the extra weight nor do I have time to eat like I did when I weighed more. A side bonus is for the first time in 22 years I can buy clothes off the rack.

Why You?

Exercise waits for no one!

Imagine for a moment, that you have just gone to the doctor and your doctor gives you the bad news: You have kidney disease. The good news is that with dialysis just a couple times weekly you will be fine.

What's the likelihood that you will tell your doc that you simply don't have enough time for dialysis? Pretty slim, I would imagine. Exercise should become this important in your life and maybe some of the surprises that do show up in routine doctor visits won't happen to you.

Each day has 24-hours in it and there are 7 days total in a week. Take away your work and sleep time and personal time is reduced significantly. If you cut out talking on the cell phone 1-hour each day or watching 1-hr of television each day you would have enough time to exercise correctly and prosper beyond your expectations.

An increase in weekly time simply is not going to happen. So, prioritize your health and 64 years of life might turn into a quality filled 74, 84 or higher. I am sure my dad would have prioritized if he had an option at this point.

So, here is a new spin on why you need to exercise; it gives the best odds for increasing your life expectancy.

Chapter 2: THE THREE TYPES OF EXERCISE TO MAINTAIN A HEALTHY LIFESTYLE AND WHY YOU NEED ALL THREE

Let's start by admitting that some of you already go to the gym and have not seen a change since you started. It's possible this is because you spend more time propping up on the equipment jawing about your day than you actually do using it for its intended purpose, improving your physique and overall health!

With that said, jawing does not count as one of the three types of exercise. If you are serious about getting fit, you have to get serious about exercise. It is possible to lose weight without exercising using a diet. The problem is you wind up sacrificing valuable lean muscle in the process and you do not strengthen your heart, lungs or build stronger bones. Instead you become skinny fat weighing a hundred pounds (hypthetical weight) but still dealing with arms that flop around when you wave at a friend. Not pretty!

The 3 types of exercise you should be doing are:

1. Cardiovascular (Metabolic Conditioning)
2. Weight Training
3. Flexibility/Stretching

1. CARDIOVASCULAR EXERCISE (Metabolic Conditioning)
STEP THIS WAY TO A LONGER LIFE!

Metabolic training? Metabolic conditioning exercises are performed with the intention of increasing the capacity and efficiency of the energy pathways to store and deliver energy for activity. Most people commonly refer to this as cardio. There are three energy pathways used to provide energy for activity, one aerobic and two anaerobic. Which of these energy pathways you should train is the source of much controversy; thus, the aerobic vs. anaerobic challenge.

AEROBIC ACTIVITY

Aerobic means in the presence of oxygen and any activity that is performed at a low to moderate intensity for more than 90 seconds. Allowing oxygen to release energy through metabolism is usually called an aerobic activity. The benefits of aerobic activity are increased cardiovascular function and decrease in body fat.

Aerobic activity is a great way for beginners to build a base of cardiovascular fitness and relieve stress that will allow them to prepare for more strenuous activity later in the KISS program.

ANAEROBIC ACTIVITY

Anaerobic means in the absence of oxygen and any activity that is performed at a medium to high intensity for less than 2 minutes, where energy is derived without oxygen, is usually called an anaerobic activity. There are two anaerobic energy pathways.

The benefits of anaerobic activity are increased cardiovascular function, increased muscle mass, improved strength, improved power, improved speed and increased aerobic capacity. Anaerobic activity requires an aerobic foundation which we are building in the first month of the program.

Physical fitness is a compromise of cardio respiratory endurance, strength, flexibility, power, speed, coordination, agility and balance. To pursue fitness excellence you must physically train to "optimize" your performance in all of the physical abilities and not "maximize" your performance in one's ability at the expense of all others. For people that do not understand that fitness is a compromise, the idea that more, longer aerobic training is indicative of a higher level of fitness is predominate. However, what they fail to realize is that by focusing on extended aerobic training exclusively, they are doing little or nothing to improve the other physical abilities needed for fitness excellence and are actually decreasing their over-all fitness level.

The human body is an amazing machine that constantly needs to be stimulated in order to improve or adapt. This is progressive overload. Combinations of anaerobic and aerobic activity will be covered in your 3-month program so that you can experience the different types of cardiovascular training and realize the benefits of each.

Calories Burned = Fat Burned = Weight Loss

Low Intensity Workouts vs. High Intensity Workouts

A high intensity workout, which is defined as exercises which push your heart rate up to 75% of its maximum or more, is infinitely better. High intensity workouts have been proven to increase metabolism and burn more calories. In fact, high intensity workouts burn 9 times more fat during exercise. The reality is that the activity that expends the greatest amount of total calories will lead to the most amount of fat burned!

HIGH INTENSITY IS NOT FOR BEGINNERS OR THOSE WITH CERTAIN HEALTH PROBLEMS.

Get clearance from a medical professional before starting any strenuous activity is written multiple times throughout this book for a reason.

The reality is that low intensity exercise burns fewer calories. To achieve the same benefits of a high intensity workout, you are going to have to exercise longer. If time is an issue then you can get more results in less time by ramping up your workout intensity. Now, I'm not saying that low intensity workouts are bad. Low intensity exercises are beneficial for warming up and cooling down before and after high intensity phases. Low intensity exercises are also good for the elderly, anyone recovering from an illness or injury, someone who is significantly overweight and out of shape, or someone who is just beginning to workout.

Low Intensity Workout vs. High Intensity Workouts:

Low Intensity Workout:
50% MHR = 7 calories per minute
90% of those calories are burning fat tissue

vs.

High Intensity Workout:
75% MHR = 14 calories per minute
60% of those calories are burning fat tissue

From the above figures, it appears that you burn more fat tissue when working at a lower intensity (90% vs. 60% from fat tissue), but these numbers are misleading.

Lets look at them another way:

Low Intensity Workout:
90% x 7 calories per minute = 6.30 fat calories burned per minute

High Intensity Workout:
60% x 14 calories per minute = 8.40 fat calories burned per minute

After you do the math, you can see that you burn a greater amount of fat tissue calories from a high intensity workout than a low intensity workout (8.4 vs. 6.3 calories burned per minute).

If you are trying to lose fat I suggest a workout that burns an average of 250 calories. Reduce your junk food calories a day by the same 250 calories (2 regular sodas) and over the course of a week you will have reduced your weight by one pound.

When I work with my clients we stay in the higher intensity work zones (anaerobic). When working on their own the intensity level drops off slightly (aerobic). This way we ensure covering the different energy pathways without overtraining. The truth is, most activities encountered in sport, work and life are a combination of all the energy pathways seamlessly flowing from one to another. My advice is to put an end to the aerobic vs. anaerobic challenge by mixing intensities. Sometimes you go easy and long, and other times you go hard and fast.

Remember, the goal is to get a longer, happier, healthier life with exercise.

2. WEIGHT LIFTING

READY TO RAISE THE BAR?

Aerobics are good for you. You should also know that you are not going to be fit unless you are weight training. Weight training is any exercise that pits your muscles against the force of gravity. Pushups, sit ups, chin ups are all examples of weight training. This is how you build bigger, stronger bones and muscles.

The combination of weight training and performing cardio allows you to burn more fat and lose less lean muscle tissue. This is because muscle burns up more fat and spares muscle tissue while you are resting. Weight training is an excellent and effective tool in changing body composition and replacing fat tissue with lean body mass.

HOW MUSCLE IS MADE AND A PLAN IS NEEDED TO BUILD IT.

HOW WEIGHT TRAINING BUILDS MUSCLE

Your muscles are made of tiny fibers bundled together. When you lift weights micro-tears are created in those fibers which later heal and grow in size, strength and firmness.

TYPES OF WEIGHTS: FREE WEIGHTS VS. WEIGHT MACHINES

Strength training can occur by the use of exercises performed with free weights or weight machines. Each has its own advantage.

Free weights have lots of versatility and one mode like the dumbbell can be used to perform hundreds of exercises. Free weights also require you to use more body control; and work more muscles at one time than machines because you have to control your body alignment throughout the movement. Free weights can be cost effective.

Machines have two major advantages over free weights. Safety, since the machines guide you through each exercises range of motion; injury chances are reduced significantly. You should always read posted instructions and warnings if you are new to exercising. Second is isolation of targeted specific muscles; useful if you need focus on one area. Once again, at the end of the day it comes back to you doing the work. Anything is possible if you simply start!

When looking at the workouts, I used dumbbells mostly. Keep in mind there are many other exercises, modes of exercise (barbells, machines, medicine balls, stability balls, etc.) but the idea behind the KISS FITNESS method is to keep it simple initially, so that you can get started on a budget with an incredible plan at your fingertips.

Weight training actually builds the size or volume of muscle that you have. At this point most females will say, "Not me!!! I don't want to look like Arnold." Rest assured, in your lifetime, you could never look like Arnold without the aid of hormone assistance (testosterone) because you simply don't make enough naturally. Plus it took him **YEARS** to look a certain way so that he could become competitive as a bodybuilder. There is a method to choosing a weight that helps you reach your goals. If you are trying to get stronger keep your reps fewer than 8; for an increase in muscle size perform 8 to 15; and if you want to improve muscular endurance then keep the repetitions 15 and over. This would be a brief overview. If you are new to exercise you should start with 12-15 repetitions.

The best answer is to combine all 3 throughout the year. My most successful one-on-one clients have benefited from lifting a heavier weight than they thought was possible to do safely. When your muscles are challenged effectively (progressive overload) and then allowed the proper amount of rest, good things are going to happen by way of toning the muscles and reducing belly fat around the waist.

A WEIGHT TRAINING PLAN

Minimal Efforts Produce Minimal Results

Every time you do a specific weight training exercise, you will perform a certain number of reps and sets and lift a specific amount of weight which will be determined by your goals, current fitness level and strength.

You might do an exercise for 3 sets of 12-15 reps at 50 pounds. Your goal will be to bring your muscles to the point of fatigue; the point at which you physically cannot do another rep with perfect form or good technique. The amount of weight chosen depends on your familiarity with the exercise or movement, your strength and your goals.

Progressing Through Sets

If you are new to exercise the first 2 sets can be performed just short of fatigue. On the last set, your goal will be to reach fatigue by the last repetition. If you still feel that you could lift more weight then start with a higher weight next workout. More experienced lifters will have an idea of how much weight to start with.

Increasing Weight, Reps or Sets

As you work on an exercise over time, it will get easier, so you will have to increase the weight, number of sets or reps to reach the same point of fatigue. This is because your nervous system is getting comfortable with this new stimulus of exercise. If you do not increase weight, sets or reps then you will plateau and your gains will decrease. Novice exercisers should always start with 12-15 reps in month 1, 10-12 reps in month 2 and 8-10 reps in month 3. You accomplish this goal by increasing your weight for each exercise. This again will allow you to experience everything that KISS FITNESS has to offer.

Tracking Your Progress

As you work through your weight training program, track your progress using the workout templates in this book. Keeping your previous information on hand when you do each workout will give you the information you need to track your progress daily. This journaling allows you to track your routine and give positive feedback when you start to see those numbers increasing as the weeks pass.

3. STRETCHING

TOUCHED YOUR TOES LATELY?

In my 22 years as an exercise enthusiast and instructor, stretching is the most widely neglected aspect of overall fitness. But, it is one of the most important aspects. If you don't believe me try and bend over and tie your shoes without having to sit down. I know some of you actually have to lie on the bed and roll onto your backs to do this.

I remember going thru security right after 9/11 in New Orleans while getting ready to board a plane to Dallas to meet with friends. There was a man probably in his mid-50's that was absolutely livid about taking off his shoes and going thru the metal detector. A few moments later, as I watched him try and put his shoes back on; I realized why he was so upset. His belly was too big and got in the way of him trying to retie his shoes, and he did not have enough flexibility to actually bend over and reach his shoes. To make matters worse, his wife did not offer to help him with the shoe laces which sent him into another level of frustration. Maybe this was all due to him being embarrassed over the obvious. Maybe, with some simple planning to get his physical life on track this could have been avoided all together.

STRETCHING TECHNIQUES

There are many different stretching techniques out there. Proprioceptive neuromuscular facilitation (PNF), contract-relax, static, dynamic and active isolated stretching (AIS) are some of the more common types. We will focus on dynamic warm-up and static techniques.

Dynamic warm-up is a series of movements that prepare your body for the demands of a workout or practice. These movements improve elasticity in the muscles preventing strains and tears; increase heart rate and respiratory rate and blood flow to the muscles. The movements take just a few minutes and also help to get you focused on the task at hand, "IMPROVEMENT." If you are having pain during the dynamic warm-up then you will want to be extra cautious during your scheduled workout.

Static stretching is an effective way to increase flexibility. It is a combination of applying pressure and isometrically contracting (without movement at the joint) a muscle in order to achieve better flexibility. It can be performed with a partner but a wall, doorway or towel can be used to facilitate the desired outcome. My one-on-one clients love this part of each session. In this book we will use a towel to help stretches of the lower body.

Keep in mind, there are other techniques out there. I just favor these. Stretches should be controlled and gentle so that you do not pop the sockets. Flexibility should be focused on the muscles being used in the workout. Warm up and cool down stretches along with their pictures and a brief description will be provided later. The dynamic warm up should be performed before every workout session.

All three types of exercise are important, right?

You now know aerobics exercise is number one in your arsenal to improve your heart and lung capacity.

You now know weight training is important because your body is made up of more than just heart tissue and lung tissue. By strengthening all of your muscles you are going to get better and be more efficient at jumping, running, walking and picking up while being less prone to injury. Weight training helps to improve your energy levels as well as reducing symptoms of stress and depression.

You now know stretching helps to keep all of these muscles flexible enough to perform the activity of choice mentioned in the aerobics and weight training components. Stretching also improves major body functions like circulation, improved posture and muscle coordination. Stretching can also help with pain or sensitive areas due to reduced range of motion and easing discomfort from your new exercise regime.

When all 3 are worked into your routine, I can guarantee you will feel better almost immediately.

An important statistic I am passing on to you is that recent studies suggest that the more arduous that exercise is the more it protected against obesity, cardiovascular disease and reduction in cognitive ability. As I have mentioned before this system will gradually build confidence and a great base for activity intensity to be increased over time. Always pay attention to what your body is telling you. Some days you are going to feel incredible and should try and push harder during the workout while other days you are not going to have the same vigor in the gym. Give what you can that day.

Chapter 3: WHAT IS YOUR LIFESTYLE PYRAMID? WHAT DOES THAT MEAN IN THE LONG TERM FOR YOUR SUCCESSFUL LIVING STRATEGY

It's important to understand how nutrition and exercise can have a positive impact on our senior years. Most of the 60 and older population are broken down into two very distinctive groups:

Group 1: the fit group that have always incorporated some level of exercise and or rigorous work daily, along with watching their food intake except maybe for special occasions. As they have aged, they are taking just a few pills a day most of which are comprised of vitamins, etc.

Group 2: the not-so-fit that have always eaten what they want, when they want and believe that they have the right to live life the way they want. They also see exercise as a waste of time and are now being held hostage by their medicine intake. A pill to control blood pressure, diabetes, anxiety, etc., is not uncommon amongst a high percentage of this population.

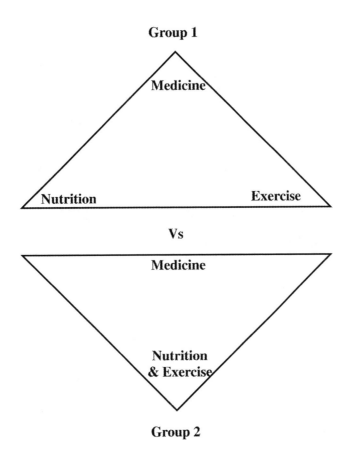

Group 1

Medicine

Nutrition   Exercise

Vs

Medicine

Nutrition
& Exercise

Group 2

So, which group do you want to be a part of? When I was 20, my mindset was similar to that of the average 20 year old, "60's old". Now that I am over 40 my thinking has changed and I want to be part of Group 1, especially since I have a family history of heart disease. Currently, the pendulum has swung in such a negative direction when it comes to childhood obesity that the 60 and older population mentioned above should be revised to include children and young adults alike.

You choose the pyramid you want to be a part of as you age! You need to get your nutrition & exercise on track or you will definitely be taking more medication as you age!

Chapter 4: THREE CRITICAL PRINCIPLES FOR A LONGER LIFE AND HEALTHIER MORE ATTRACTIVE YOU

PRINCIPLE #1: CONSISTENCY

The Best Looking People in the Gym are in the gym!

Look around the gym, what do all the people with the best bodies have in common? They are in the gym on a regular basis; you see them every time you go. Some may socialize a lot, others may workout hard and head home right away, some may have trainers, and others may be loners who keep to themselves. No matter what style of training they use, what they all do is find a way to get into the gym and train hard consistently. If you want great results, you need to be committed and consistent in your workouts. Forget dietary supplements or any other infomercials that promise you a swimsuit calendar body without breaking a sweat. If you want to make major changes you have to earn it. You may be asking yourself, "How much time is necessary?" It varies from person to person. We all have busy lives with work, school, kids, etc. If you want to obtain that perfect physique, you have to prioritize your life to find the time to achieve your goals.

How long does it take to morph your body? A better question is, "How long does it take to change your life?" That is what you are really doing. Life changes are what lead to body and fitness changes. With the exception of plastic surgery, you cannot physically change your body; you can only pressure it through lifestyle, diet, exercise, and supplementation. Your goal is to change your habits and choices, and pressure your body into building lean muscle and shredding body fat. You are going to get the tools to attack your body and rebuild it; the question is, will you use them? This program is a progressive workout and education which will morph your body and lifestyle in 3 months, if you apply it. Think about it: 3 phases, 12 weeks to a new you.

If you work through this program, I can promise you that you will see results in the mirror and you will feel better about yourself. How can I promise you this? You do not need the greatest program ever to achieve results. You need a progressive program that changes at strategic times and forces you to adapt; all the while checking your progress and tweaking it whenever needed so you can continue to get results. In 3 months, we are going to teach you how to adapt your program to keep getting results and bust through plateaus. Who do you want to see in the mirror 3 months from now?

Lucky People and Reality

Yes, we know some people are gifted with amazing looks and great bodies, but these are not the people you need to imitate. It's ok to be inspired or motivated, but realizing your individual potential and desires are most important. Each of us has a physical gift that someone else admires (really!!!). So, let's focus on what you can achieve in your own skin. You need to find people who have been in your shoes and have made it to the next level. The question, "will this work for me?" is answered at the end of the 3 months. We are just talking 3 months of commitment. That is what this program is about.

PRINCIPLE #2: TECHNIQUE

Posture During Exercise

Though ignoring good form and technique might allow you to lift heavier weight, it will actually slow down your progress and increase your chances of injury.

Basic knowledge is essential before you jump into a gym. This will keep you safe and increase your progress. Essentially, you will get more bangs for your training buck if you start off with a good foundation. The first month will be spent on building your core foundation.

The basis for a good lifting technique is having a strong posture during the exercise. You always use controlled movements both when raising and lowering the weight. Keep your spine straight when lifting or pulling a weight. If you feel like you are starting to arch the back simply engage your abs and try and tuck your tailbone under you. Do not hunch the shoulders or round them. Think of keeping your ears away from your shoulders. Never allow your joints to lock out; this can cause injury when applying heavier weights. Most important and sometimes forgotten, **BREATHE!** Inhale as you lift a weight and exhale as you bring it back to the starting position.

Most of us either have ourselves or know of someone with severely rounded shoulders. As a young teenager I had a 6 inch growth spurt between 7th grade and 8th grade. My muscles at this point were not trained or strong enough to support the bones and so began my slumping forward at the shoulders. Every time my father saw me in this posture he would make me stand up against the wall in our family room with the back of my head touching the wall, followed by my shoulder blades, butt, calves and finally my feet. As my career started to take off, I used this same technique to help clients that were suffering from headaches, shoulder discomfort and lower back pain. Since most of us have computer stations that have not been set up properly from an ergonomic standpoint these symptoms are common. By looking at the picture below you can see the difference in the correct and incorrect posture while standing or sitting.

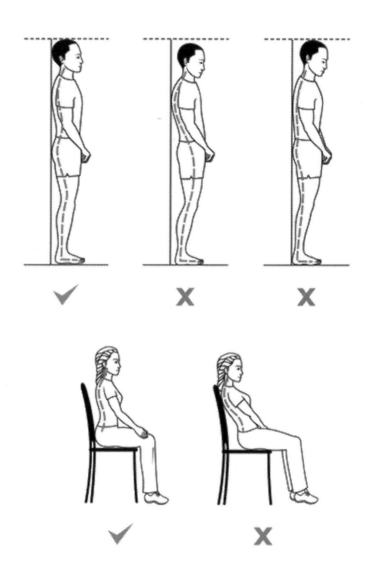

RANGE OF MOTION

You should go through a full range of motion with each exercise as long as your joints allow it. If you feel joint pain during an exercise, STOP! Lifting weights is not supposed to cause pain in joints. Either adjust the exercise or seek medical attention if pain persists. Pushing through pain only leads to injuries and months away from the gym in rehabilitation. What do you think your physique will look like then?

PRINCIPLE #3: PROGRESS

You do not have to be perfect with your training to get results, but you do have to be progressive and maintain an appropriate level of intensity. I have had clients that obsess over every calorie they eat. They can tell you the fat, protein and carbohydrate in almost every food known. However, they fail to record their workouts and check their progress. This is fine if you already have the physique you want, but not if you are trying to realize change in your best body possible. The effort and planning needed to make major changes in your body and life are far greater than those needed to maintain it. We have one defining question that decides for us whether or not we have had a good workout; ___did I Improve?___ It is ok to be sore or tired, but that does not necessarily mean muscle growth and fat loss. Simply put: if you get better in the gym, you'll look better outside the gym. If you are serious about making a change, you need to record your progress and strive to improve each time you workout. How you feel about the workout is important but is secondary to the actual results of the workout. Not sure yet? Get into your underwear and take a look in the mirror. The mirror never lies. I tell everyone this answer in response to the question how much weight should I lose.

REST

Not only is a hard work out necessary for optimal performance, but also resting your body is important. When you work out the body, muscle fibers are torn and its energy systems are depleted. This causes the body to adapt by rebuilding better and stronger muscles with improved energy systems, as long as the body has the time and nutrients to accomplish the task. Think of it as building a garden. You can keep tilling up the land (tearing down muscle fibers), but if you never plant the seeds (feed your body nutrients) and give them time to grow (rest periods) you will never harvest your crop (accomplish your fitness goal). You need to work out hard and challenge your body so it has a reason to improve, but then you also have to feed and rest your body in order for it to make those improvements. This is why you will see rest or recovery days during your exercising week. This does not mean you need to plop yourself on the couch and pass countless hours gaming on the computer (remember the poor posture speech). Instead, look to incorporate something fun outside of the gym.

I started playing golf recently as a way to get away from the gym. This allows my time in the gym to remain exciting. If you worry about losing your edge and getting back to the old mind set, continue to exercise just stay away from anything that causes you to be taxed at the end.

WHEN TO INCREASE / NOT INCREASE THE WEIGHT?

When do I increase weight? Simply put, whenever you have mastered it. Month 1 of your KISS workout has many exercises in which you are scheduled to perform 2-4 sets of each exercise. If you can only perform 1 set of your chosen number of reps (15 for example if you are building muscle size) and 1 set of 6 on the following set, then you are not ready to up the weight. As soon as you can properly perform 2-3 full sets of 15 repetitions, add more weight in the next workout and start over. Continue this cycle until month 1 is complete and it is time to move on to the next month of training.

To experience the full effect of KISS Fitness in month 1, choose a weight that you can lift safely and with proper form 12-15 reps; month 2 choose a weight that can be lifted 10-12 reps and in month 3 choose a weight that can be lifted 8-10 reps or for 60-seconds. This last offering is explained later in more detail.

There is one pitfall that I see novice and expert gym goers alike make; they skip ahead in their program because the workout appears to be easy. If your weights are not heavy enough to achieve measureable results each month, then add more weight. If the increase in weight makes you feel apprehensive or nervous about injury, then add another set of each exercise at the current controllable weight. It will always come back to you putting the needed time and effort in the gym. With 22 years of trial and error I can guarantee the success of the workouts. Remember that like many endeavors in your life you are in control.

Chapter 5: HOW THE PLAN WORKS

PRE-PROGRAM TESTS:

Below I have listed some tests for you to take prior to starting the program. It is a great idea to get clearance from your general physician plus base line tests like cholesterol (HDL/LDL), blood sugar, etc. You are going to improve with these workouts and this program. Wouldn't it be great to know by how much improvement was made? If you do not want the hassle of going thru your general physician, most cities in the US have independent labs which will perform these tests for around $40. All you need to do is bring in the list below. Obviously, if you are having a mammogram test performed you would not let a lab tech perform it. You would see a specialist. Anything blood related can be done at a lab with almost instant results.

MEDICAL TESTS FOR WOMEN

How healthy are you? During your 40s is a great time to assess the current state of your health, correct the abuses of your past, and prepare your body for the next four, five, or even six decades of your life!

Your doctor can help by checking you for problems that can rob you of your health. Here's a list of the basic tests women should ask for.

> **BLOOD SUGAR.** Decades of eating the wrong food (think chocolate, hot dogs, fries -- you get the picture) plus weight gain plus hormone changes may have overworked your poor pancreas.
>
> **BREAST EXAM AND MAMMOGRAM**. You're probably checking your breasts at home regularly, (you better) and your doctor does an exam annually. Decide when to start with your doctor.
>
> **BLOOD PRESSURE.** You can lower your blood pressure through diet, exercise, and medication. It's worth the effort. Lower blood pressure is a key factor in longevity.
>
> **CHOLESTEROL PROFILE.** Take it to heart: this simple blood test can save your life. One in five Americans has high cholesterol, a condition that leads to heart attacks or strokes. Diseases that claim a life every 33 seconds!

PELVIC EXAM AND PAP. Yes, you still need these, especially if you're sexually active. Ten minutes of mild discomfort once every one to three years pays big dividends in protecting you from cancer and sexually transmitted diseases.

MOLES. Years of getting "a healthy tan" can lead to something not so healthy - skin cancer. Luckily, most skin cancers are curable.

CHECK YOUR EYES. Having trouble reading or working at the computer? Be sure to get your eyes examined regularly: every one to two years to check for common problems like presbyopia, glaucoma and macular degeneration. Go more often if you have vision problems.

IMMUNIZATIONS. Ask your doctor if you need a tetanus booster shot, and whether you should consider a flu shot.

Being overweight puts you at high risk for developing a number of diseases, including diabetes and heart disease. Again, take off your clothes and stand in front of the mirror if you think you are "in-shape!"

MEDICAL TESTS FOR MEN

BLOOD PRESSURE. High blood pressure can cause serious organ damage or death. But screening for it is easy and reliable. Blood pressure check is part of most routine doctor's visits.

CHOLESTEROL. Start checking age 35 and up. It also recommends screening for men 20 and up if they have other risk factors for heart disease. Risk factors are things like diabetes or a family history of heart disease or high cholesterol. Cholesterol levels are less likely to increase after age 65.

COLORECTAL CANCER. Colon cancer kills more than 56,000 people every year. But the CDC says that nearly 60% of those deaths could be prevented if everyone was screened properly and treated appropriately. It is strongly recommended of all men (and women) age 50 and up for colorectal cancer. People at higher risk may need to be screened at a younger age. This includes people who have a close relative who had colorectal polyps or cancer or who have inflammatory bowel disease.

IMMUNIZATIONS. Immunity can fade over time, and vaccine recommendations change over the years. For men over 50, a tetanus booster is recommended every 10 years, flu shots are suggested every year.

PROSTATE CANCER. Prostate cancer screenings are among the most controversial medical tests today. While the PSA can detect prostate cancer in its early stages, it can also return many false positives. I suggest talking to your doctor about the relation between prostate cancer, age, and family history. Then you can decide together whether to take the PSA. The PSA is most likely to benefit men aged 50 to 70. It can also be beneficial if you are over 45 and are at increased risk.

DIABETES. I recommend diabetes screening for adults who have high blood pressure or cholesterol issues.

SKIN CANCER. The American Academy of Dermatologists suggests a monthly self-exam to look for irregular moles. A trip to a dermatologist once a year for a complete skin exam is recommended.

TESTICULAR CANCER. Testicular cancer mainly affects young men, ages 20 to 39. Though testicular cancer is rare, it is curable if detected early.

PROTECTING YOUR EYES. Having trouble reading or working at the computer? Be sure to get your eyes examined regularly; every one to two years to check for common problems like presbyopia, glaucoma and macular degeneration. Go more often if you have vision problems.

This year, give yourself the gift that keeps on giving. Schedule a visit to your dentist, and call your doctor to see if there are important tests you should take not listed here. By investing an hour or so with the doctor now, you may be able to add years to your life.

PAPERWORK

Now that you have these baseline numbers you are ready to start with the workouts.

You need to take the 2 workouts from month 1 and make 6 copies of each and put them in a binder along with one copy of your warm up movements and static stretches. You have 2 different workouts because we have different angles or exercises that we work in the different workouts. You make 6 copies of each workout because you are going to perform these 2 workouts 6 times each. I want you to master each movement before we move on to month 2. After making copies, decide which days you are going to work out. It is important to keep in mind that you need at least 24 hours of rest in between similar workouts. So establish a Monday, Wednesday, Friday workout or Tuesday, Thursday, Saturday and commit.

TIME COMMITTMENT

If you are going to perform strength training and cardio on separate days then it should take between 20-45 minutes 6 times a week. If you are doing weights, cardio and core on the same day then it will take longer, but you will be in the gym fewer days.

Cardio and Core Workouts can be performed on opposite days from strength days and a sample week of this formula is listed below.

Example: Week 1 of Months 1 and 2

Monday	Tuesday	Wednesday	Thursday	Friday	Saturday	Sunday
Workout 1	Cardio & Core	Workout 2	Cardio & Core	Workout 1	Cardio & Core	OFF

Week 2 of month 1 would start off with Workout 2. This is the bases that KISS uses for its first 2-months, but it can be manipulated to fit your schedule. What is most important is that you accomplish the total volume of exercises. The only rule is not to perform two or more weight training workouts in subsequent days. There needs to be at least one day off between workouts 2 and 3 to avoid overstressing your body whenever possible.

Month 3 will look slightly different.

Example: Week 1

Monday	Tuesday	Wednesday	Thursday	Friday	Saturday	Sunday
Workout 1	Workout 2	Cardio & Core	Workout 3	Workout 4	Cardio & Core	OFF

RECORD

Each day you go into the gym, record the weights and reps that you do for each exercise along with the cardio work (calories burned, distance travelled or overall strides per minute and time). When you finish all of your workout days of training and cardio you will be able to look back and get some understanding of what you have accomplished in month one of the program. Recording your progress is crucial to long-term success. This will also let you know that it is time to leave month 1 and move on to month 2 when all 12 copies have been used up.

In month 2 you are going to perform three different workouts four times before moving on to month 3. Use the same established workout days from month-1 (Monday, Wednesday, Friday or Tuesday, Thursday, Saturday). If you have to go multiple days in a row, this is ok because the workouts are broken down into more work and fewer body parts being worked than in month 1. It is most important to get the work in. Our daily lives are not perfect, therefore a Monday, Wednesday, Friday schedule may not be possible. **Just make it work!**

Your 3 different workouts will be broken down into an Upper Body Pull Workout, Lower Body Workout and Upper Body Push Workout. We are going to introduce interval cardio this month. Watch as your physical conditioning jumps to the next level and physical changes begin.

Month 3 will have 2 workouts where each workout will be performed twice each week. You will make 8 copies of each. We will use a 2 on / 1 off approach where you will work out 2 days in a row and rest 1 day and then start over. Again, if you have to work out multiple days in a row do it. Just do not miss the week entirely.

Intensity this last month will be high, high, high. The cardio will be included in the workout instead of after. This method is called is super-circuit training or short burst training. If you would like to perform "recovery" cardio on the off days do it. Just keep in mind that your goal is to recover. Your heart rate should not rise so much that you would have trouble providing an answer to a question if someone asked one.

Chapter 6: MONTH BY MONTH

With each program you will notice that there are pictures of each exercise that shows a starting and finishing position so that you can see how to perform the exercise properly. So, instead of carrying a clunky book or magazine, you simply bring in your binder and a pencil to write down your results. By the end of the month you should have mastered each movement and as a result, built the first level of your new body foundation.

For each month you will get a brief description of the desired outcome and will see a few terms like anaerobic. In the back of the book there is a glossary of terms that you can always refer to if needed.

Below is an overview of what the 3 months will look like:

KISS Overview

Weeks	Monday	Tuesday	Wednesday	Thursday	Friday	Saturday	Sunday
1	Weights	Cardio & Core	Weights	Cardio & Core	Weights	Cardio & Core	OFF
2	Weights	Cardio & Core	Weights	Cardio & Core	Weights	Cardio & Core	OFF
3	Weights	Cardio & Core	Weights	Cardio & Core	Weights	Cardio & Core	OFF
4	Weights	Cardio & Core	Weights	Cardio & Core	Weights	Cardio & Core	OFF
5	Weights	Cardio & Core	Weights	Cardio & Core	Weights	Cardio & Core	OFF
6	Weights	Cardio & Core	Weights	Cardio & Core	Weights	Cardio & Core	OFF
7	Weights	Cardio & Core	Weights	Cardio & Core	Weights	Cardio & Core	OFF
8	Weights	Cardio & Core	Weights	Cardio & Core	Weights	Cardio & Core	OFF
9	Weights	Weights	Cardio & Core	Weights	Weights	Cardio & Core	OFF
10	Weights	Weights	Cardio & Core	Weights	Weights	Cardio & Core	OFF
11	Weights	Weights	Cardio & Core	Weights	Weights	Cardio & Core	OFF
12	Weights	Weights	Cardio & Core	Weights	Weights	Cardio & Core	OFF

MONTH 1

In month-1, we are going to build a new attitude towards exercise. We are using a routine which will burn a lot of calories at a low intensity level. The idea is to build core strength. This phase fixes weak links while preparing the body for the more demanding workouts in the following phases. The focal points this month are: proper nutrition and body fat loss.

The routine uses a circuit method of training in which you will perform one set of each exercise before moving on to the next exercise in the workout. After you have made it thru each exercise once, you can go back and start over for the prescribed number of sets. You should note that the exercises are broken down into lower body exercises and upper body exercises on the same workout. The rest periods are very short, which allows you to keep working mainly in the metabolic system throughout the workout. Workouts are not going to last long.

It is important for you to stick as close to the rest periods as possible so you can attain maximum results from the program. At the end of each circuit of exercises rest up to 90-seconds if you need to before starting the second round. But, if you do not need a lot of rest time then by all means carry on. This means as little socializing outside of general pleasantries while working out. If you feel fine then shorten the rest period.

For cardio, it does not matter what training method you use: running, swimming, cycle classes, body bar, kickboxing, etc. The goal is to keep your heart rate elevated for more than 20 minutes straight. If you do so then you are on the right track. How do you tell if you are working hard enough? It all comes down to one simple question. Just ask yourself, "Did I improve on this workout from the last workout?" Did I walk farther, burn more calories, etc.?

The success of every workout, whether it is a cardio day or a weight day, can be attributed to the answer of that question. So, pick a type or mode of exercise you like and can perform for at least 20-30 minutes straight. Once again, no phones or too much socializing!

NOTE: This is where I feel classes are a great strategy because you can be social without having to speak and you will stay in a productive heart rate level.

It is important to follow each component of your exercise experience to the letter. First do a warm-up, next the strength training, cardio training followed by a brief cool-down stretch period.

MONTH 1

MONTH 1: GOALS
o   Establish foods that are healthy that you enjoy eating
o   Meals are spread out over 5 balanced calorie meals
o   3-4 sets X reps per exercise you choose based on goal
o   Weights 3 times a week focusing on building symmetry
o   Rest breaks are short between sets
o   Cardio 3 times a week over 20 minutes with elevated heart rate

WORKOUT LOG				
RESISTANCE TRAINING WORKOUT 1/ MONTH1				
Exercise	Sets 4	Reps	Rest	Week (_)
Dumbbell Bench Press				
Dumbbell Split Leg Squat (lunge)				
Dumbbell Bent Over Row				
Stability Ball Supine Leg Curl				
Dumbbell Standing Arm Curl				

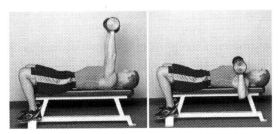

Dumbbell Chest Press

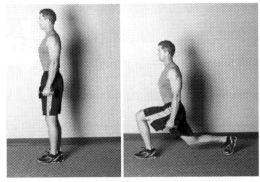

Dumbbell Split Leg Squat (Lunge)

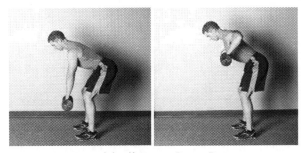

Dumbbell Bent Over Row

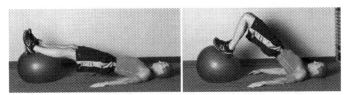

Stability Ball Supine Leg Curl

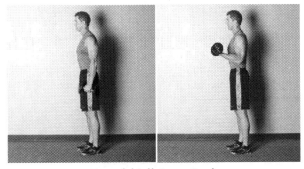

Dumbbell Arm Curl

Dumbbell Chest Press:

To do the chest press with dumbbells, lie on your back with a dumbbell in each hand. Hold your upper arms perpendicular to your body and your forearms perpendicular to the floor. Slowly press the weights upward until your elbows are almost straight. Your hands will face forward throughout entire movement.

Dumbbell Split Leg Squat:

Stand with dumbbells at sides. Stand with feet far apart, one-foot forward and other foot behind. Squat down by flexing knee and hip of front leg until knee of rear leg is almost in contact with floor. Return to original standing position by extending hip and knee of forward leg. Repeat.

Dumbbell Bent Over Row:

Stand with legs shoulder width apart with a dumbbell in each hand, palms facing the body. Bend over at the waist keeping the back straight. Eyes should be just in front of your toes if you look down. Slowly bring DB's up and to the outside of the chest. Shoulder blades should be squeezed together. After max contraction lower hands back to starting position.

Stability Ball Leg Curl:

Start on your back with heels on top, center of ball. Slowly squeeze your butt and lift hips off ground and pull heels toward the butt. Keeping butt tight slowly extend heels back to starting position.

Dumbbell Arm Curl:

Position two dumbbells at sides, palms facing in, and arms straight. With elbows at sides, raise one dumbbell and rotate forearm until forearm is vertical and palm faces shoulder. Lower to original position and repeat with opposite arm. Continue to alternate between sides.

WORKOUT LOG				
RESISTANCE TRAINING WORKOUT 2/ MONTH 1				
Exercise	Sets 4	Reps	Rest	Week (_)
Dumbbell Overhead Press				
Dumbbell Step Down Lunge (Curtsey Lunge)				
Close Grip Pull Down				
Dumbbell Bent Knee Romanian Dead Lift				
DB Skull Crusher				

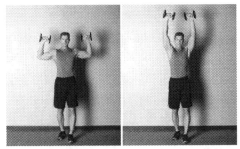

Dumbbell Overhead Press

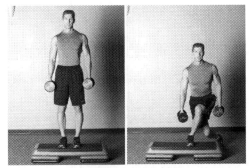

Dumbbell Step Down Lunge (Curtsey Lunge)

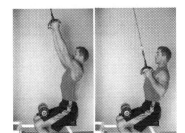

Close Grip Pull Down

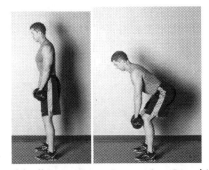

Dumbbell Bent Knee Romanian Dead Lift

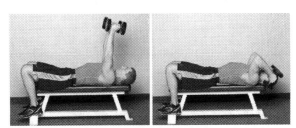

Dumbbell Skull Crusher

Dumbbell Overhead Press:

Hold one dumbbell in each hand at shoulder height with the elbows pointed downward and to the sides. Exhale as you drive both dumbbells overhead until the elbows are fully extended. Keep the head upright and in a neutral position. At no time should you bend it forward. Slowly lower the dumbbells to the starting position while inhaling.

Dumbbell Step Down Lunge (curtsey lunge):

Stand with both feet on a box or elevated area. With dumbbell in each hand step down and outside of left leg with the right foot; foot should lightly touch floor. Pause for one count and slowly apply pressure into left floor which is still on box and bring right foot back to starting position. Switch sides and repeat.

Close Grip Pull Down:

Sit with hips right under the pads. Take a slightly less than shoulder-width, underhand grip (palms facing you) on the bar. Start with arms straight over your head; pull the bar down to your chest. Puff your chest up to meet the bar and try to squeeze your shoulder blades together behind your back. Let the bar up slowly then repeat.

Dumbbell Romanian Dead lift:

Grab a pair of dumbbells using a pronated (palms facing body) grip with hands a little wider than shoulder width. Lower the dumbbells by pushing the hips back, only slightly bending the knees, unlike when squatting. The finished position will be when you can no longer push your rear end back and dumbbells are in the knee area. A nice pulling sensation should be felt behind the legs. Return to starting position. **Tip:** The movement should not be fast but steady and under control.

Dumbbell Skull Crusher:

Lie on bench and position dumbbells overhead with arms extended. Lower dumbbells by bending elbow until they are at sides of head. Elbows should remain pointed towards ceiling. Extend arm and repeat.

Cardio Workout Month 1					
Week ( )					
Exercise		Time	Speed	Intensity	Distance
Base Cardio (Any continuous cardiovascular exercise)	Day 1	20 min			
Base Cardio (Any continuous cardiovascular exercise)	Day 2	20 min			
Base Cardio (Any continuous cardiovascular exercise)	Day 3	20 min			

Core Workout Month 1			
Exercise	**Sets** **4**	**Time** **30-60 sec**	**Week (_)**
Plank			
Side Plank			
Straight Leg Raise			

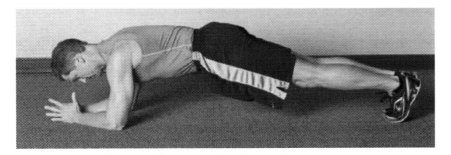

Plank

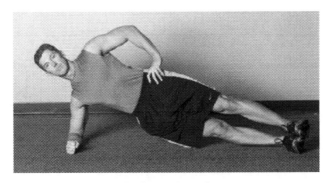

Side Plank

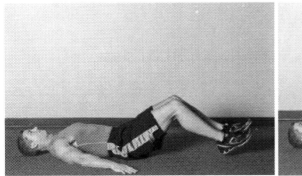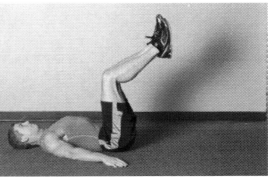

Straight Leg Raise

Plank:

Start by lying face down on the ground. Place your elbows and forearms underneath your chest. Prop yourself up to form a bridge using your toes and forearms. Maintain a flat back and do not allow your hips to sag towards the ground.

Side Plank:

Lift your body of the ground and balance on one forearm and the side of your foot. Contract your abdominals and relax your shoulders and breathe. If you need an easier version simply bend knees to 90 degrees with feet pointed behind you. Once again you would lift your body off ground maintaining balance on one forearm, knee closest to ground and side of your foot.

Straight Leg Raise:

Hands should be at sides of body or slightly away from the body. Keeping legs straight and together, back flat, lift legs upward until they are straight above hips; lower down to starting position slowly and with control (but do not allow feet to touch the ground between reps) to complete one rep. If this is too hard simply bend at the knees to relieve stress in abdominals and lower back.

MONTH 2

The workout is going to be a muscle building workout. It is the bodybuilding part of this program meant to increase muscle and metabolism while shedding tons of unsightly fat. The intensity level is moderate but the volume of training is high, which makes recovery from training important in this phase. You are going to need a high quality nutrition habit in order to stick with the amount of work in this routine.

Your 3 workouts will be performed each week to ensure adequate recovery. They will be broken down into an Upper Body Pull, Lower Body and Upper Body Push. This months' core work will be performed the same as in month 1, but you will be performing the next level of each move and on the same day as cardio.

The weekends should be taken off completely unless you start your workout on Tuesday. Then you will take off Sunday and Monday from the gym or something away from the gym should be substituted instead. Perform 4 sets of each exercise before moving to the next exercise, rest 30-seconds between each set.

In this phase, you will be introduced to interval cardio. For example, if you perform 30-minutes of cardio at least part of it will be at a high level while the other is spent recovering. So you want to push yourself for a set amount of time followed by an amount of recovery time which is determined by how long it takes you to catch your breath. For the beginner, you might want to try 60 seconds of work followed by 60 seconds of recovery. For the fit individual, you might want to go 60 seconds hard followed by 30 seconds of recovery. You decide. Just remember, improve every time.

MONTH 2: GOALS
- Training and nutrition are both keys
- Aim to consume 1 gallon of water a day
- Shoot for increasing weights each workout
- Weights 3 times weekly
- Rest 30 seconds between sets
- Complete all sets for each exercise before moving to next exercise
- Learn to enjoy interval cardio

WORKOUT LOG				
WORKOUT 1/ MONTH 2 UPPER BODY PULL				
Exercise	Sets 4	Reps	Rest	Week ( )
Wide Grip Pull Down				
1-Arm Row Cable Row				
Dumbbell Lateral Raise				
Dumbbell High Pull				
Dumbbell Biceps Curl				

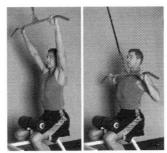

Wide Grip Pull Down

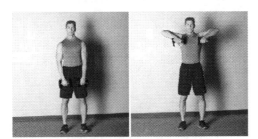

1-Arm Row Cable Row

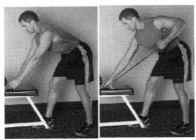

Dumbbell Lateral Raise

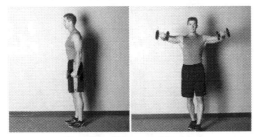

Dumbbell High Pull

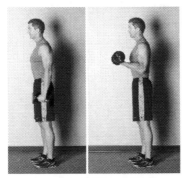

Dumbbell Bicep Curl

Wide Grip Pull Down:

Sit with hips right under the pads. Take a slightly wider than shoulder-width, overhand grip (palms facing away) on the bar. Start with arms straight over your head; pull the bar down to your chest. Puff your chest up to meet the bar and try to squeeze your shoulder blades together behind your back. Let the bar up slowly then repeat.

1-Arm Cable Row:

Stand to side of rotating pulley at medium to low height. Place hand shoulder height or slightly lower on support bar with arm straight. Place foot nearest supporting arm forward with knee slightly bent and opposite foot back. Grasp cable stirrup with one hand allowing shoulder to be pulled forward under weight on cable. Pull cable attachment to side of torso while pulling shoulder back, arching spine, and pushing chest forward. Return until arm is extended and shoulder is pulled forward. Repeat and continue with opposite arm.

Dumbbell Lateral Raise:

Grab two dumbbells and stand with your feet shoulder width apart. Hold the dumbbells in front of your thighs with your palms facing in. Draw in the belly button and maintain proper posture throughout the entire exercise. While keeping your arms straight, lift the dumbbells outwards until your arms are perpendicular to your body. Slowly return the weight to the starting position.

Dumbbell High Pull:

Start in a standing position holding the dumbbells in front of you. Pulling with you arms, bring the dumbbells to shoulder height. Lower the dumbbells and return to the starting position. Elbows should remain higher than hands throughout movement.

Dumbbell Biceps Curl:

Position two dumbbells at sides, palms facing in, and arms straight. With elbows at sides, raise one dumbbell and rotate forearm until forearm is vertical and palm faces shoulder. Lower to original position and repeat with opposite arm. Continue to alternate between sides.

WORKOUT LOG				
WORKOUT 2/ MONTH 2 LOWER BODY				
Exercise	Sets 4	Reps	Rest	Week (_)
Barbell Squat				
Dumbbell Travelling Lunge				
Cable Abduction (Outer Thigh)				
Dumbbell Bent Knee Deadlift				
Dumbbell Standing Heel Raise				

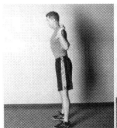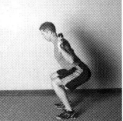

Barbell Squat

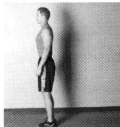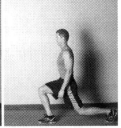

Dumbbell Travelling Lunge

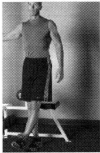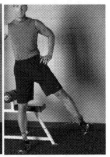

Cable Abduction (Outer Thigh)

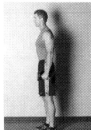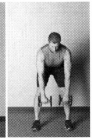

Dumbbell Bent Knee Dead Lift

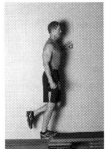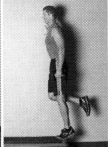

Dumbbell Standing Heel Raise

Barbell Squat:

Barbell should be resting behind the neck just below the upper back muscles. Bend knees forward while allowing hips to bend back behind, keeping back straight and knees pointed same direction as feet. Descend until thighs are just past parallel to floor. Extend knees and hips until legs are straight. Return and repeat.

Dumbbell Travelling Lunge:

Stand with dumbbells at sides. Step forward with first leg landing on a soft foot. Lower body by flexing knee and hip of front leg until knee of rear leg is almost in contact with floor. Stand on forward leg with assistance of rear leg. Lunge forward with opposite leg. Repeat by alternating lunge with opposite legs.

Cable Abduction (outer thigh):

Stand in front of low pulley facing to one side. Attach cable cuff to far ankle. Step out away from stack and grasp ballet bar. Stand on near foot and allow far leg to cross in front. Move leg to opposite side of low pulley by abduction hip. Return and repeat. Turn around and continue with opposite leg.

Dumbbell Bent Knee Deadlift:

Stand in an upright position while holding dumbbells at your sides. Lower the dumbbells down toward the floor by first sitting your hips back; bend your knees and torso until your reach just above the floor. Keep your back flat and your head in a neutral position throughout the movement. Make sure you keep the dumbbells near your sides. Don't let them swing out in front of your body. Return to start position.

Dumbbell Standing Heel Raise:

Grasp dumbbell in one hand to side. Position toes and balls of feet on calf block or elevated surface with arches and heels extending off. Place hand on support for balance. Lift other leg to rear by bending knee. Raise heel by extending ankle as high as possible. Lower heel by bending ankle until calf is stretched. Repeat and continue with opposite leg.

WORKOUT LOG				
WORKOUT 3/ MONTH 2 UPPER BODY PUSH				
Exercise	Sets 4	Reps	Rest	Week (_)
Dumbbell Incline Chest Press				
Dumbbell Alternating Overhead Press				
Body Weight Push-ups with Feet Elevated				
Dumbbell Chest Fly				
Dumbbell Straight Arm Lateral Raise				

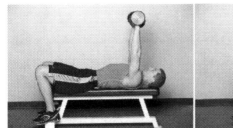

Dumbbell Incline Chest Press

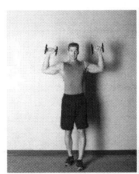

Dumbbell Alternating Overhead Press

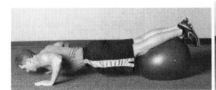

Body Weight Push-ups with Feet Elevated

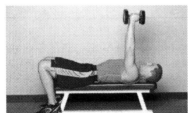

Dumbbell Chest Fly

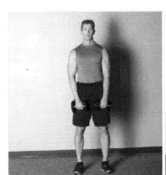

Dumbbell Straight Arm Lateral Raise

Dumbbell Incline Chest Press:

Sit down on incline bench with dumbbells resting on lower thigh. Kick (using knee) weights to shoulders and lean back; position dumbbells to sides of chest with upper arm under each dumbbell. Press dumbbells up with elbows at sides until arms are extended and hands forward. Lower weight to sides of upper chest until slight stretch is felt in chest or shoulder. Repeat. ***Image shows flat chest press. Apply incline level to your comfort.**

Dumbbell Alternating Overhead Press:

Grab a pair of dumbbells and raise them overhead with palm forward (if you have a shoulder problem you can lift with palms facing each other). Slowly lower one hand until it reaches just below ears and then press dumbbell back to starting position. Alternate sides and repeat.

Push-ups with Feet Elevated on Stability Ball:

Assume start position as shown by placing stability ball under the front of legs at the shin level. Bend at elbows to lower your body down toward the floor and then slowly press up to starting position. If this is to easy simply walk your legs further out on the ball until feet are in center of ball.

Dumbbell Chest Fly:

To do the chest fly with dumbbells, lie on your back with a dumbbell in each hand. Hold your upper arms perpendicular to your body and your forearms perpendicular to the floor. Slowly press the weights upward until your elbows are straight. Your palms should face each other at all times.

Dumbbell Straight Arm Lateral Raise:

Lean forward slightly, with flexed knees and slightly rounded back. When lifting the dumbbells, your hands and arms should not be at your sides but at roughly 10 o' clock and 2 o' clock. Try to keep the hand as parallel to the floor as possible. Lean more or less to direct the focus to the lateral head. It is **IMPORTANT** that you keep the elbow just slightly bent or unlocked, to minimize the stress on the elbow joint. Let comfort be your guide as to the correct amount of bend. This exercise is not a power movement.

Cardio Workout Month 2					
Week ( )					
Exercise		Time	Speed	Intensity	Distance
Any Cardio	Day 1	20-30 min			
30 Seconds Fast/ 30 Seconds Recovery					
Any Cardio	Day 2	20-30 min			
30 Seconds Fast/ 30 Seconds Recovery					
Any Cardio	Day 3	20-30 min			
30 Seconds Fast/ 30 Seconds Recovery					

Core Workout Month 2			
Exercise	**Sets** **4**	**Time** **30-60 sec**	**Week (_)**
Plank w/ 3 Contact Points			
Side Plank with Feet Elevated			
Low Back Extension on Floor			

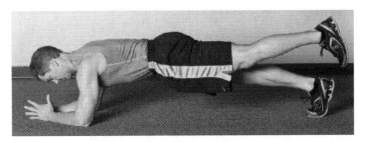

Plank with 3 Contact Points

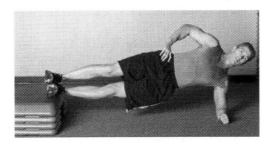

Side Plank with Feet Elevated

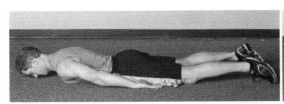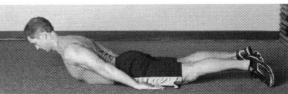

Low Back Extension on Floor

Plank w/ 3 Contact Points:

Start by lying face down on the ground. Place your elbows and forearms underneath your chest. Prop yourself up to form a bridge using your toes and forearms. Maintain a flat back and do not allow your hips to sag towards the ground. From this starting position you can either lift 1-foot or 1-hand. Your goal is to extend it away from the body instead of trying to lift it higher. This will help keep body in perfect alignment. Feel free to alternate slowly between a foot and then a leg on one side of body and then opposite side of body.

Side Plank w/ Feet Elevated:

 Lift your body of the ground and balance on one forearm and the sides of your feet elevated on a step, bench or stability ball. Contract your abdominals and relax your shoulders and breathe.

Low Back (prone) Extension on Floor:

With arms at side, palms down, contract the pelvis and legs while slowly lifting the torso off the floor. Be sure to keep the chin tucked during the movement to prevent neck strain while keeping contact of the pelvis and legs with the floor. Hold this position for a count of 2-4, then return to the starting position.

MONTH 3

You will be introduced to Short Burst Training (SBT). It is a unique concept of mixing cardio and weights in one seamless workout. This type of training is high intensity throughout the workout. At this point if you have followed the program then you are ready for this last month of our commitment. This is where major physical changes will become obvious. It will be great!

SHORT BURST TRAINING "MY STYLE OF TRAINING"

High-intensity, short duration interval workouts are a new frontier in fitness and sports training.

When you are a sports fan, it does not matter if you like basketball, football, track and field or ice skating-you're sure to admire the performance of an athlete that works inconceivably hard to achieve greatness. I have been moved a number of times to go instantly to the gym and try something new.

Short burst training (SBT) is a variation of circuit training, using circuit training with high-intensity and short duration exercises interspersed with brief periods of lower intensity movement. Exercisers go all out for 30-60 seconds before entering recovery phase. This pattern is repeated throughout the workout. The intent is to utilize the anaerobic (without oxygen) energy system, long thought to be the arena of sprinters and court athletes whose movements are too brief and powerful to engage the oxygen pathways of the cardiovascular system.

Cardiovascular exercise follows the short burst of anaerobic exercise and helps to buffer the waste products caused by the intensity of the movement. The primary fuel used is carbohydrate with stored fat kicking in later.

Traditional aerobic training is praised for improving the body's efficiency at burning stored fat once activity stops, a term called excess post-exercise oxygen consumption (EPOC). Trainers call it the after-burn. More and more studies are showing that SBT is even better at burning more stored up fat (fuel) for as much as 24-hours after exercise has ceased. The research is not saying that we should sell our stationary bike or treadmill. For those of us that want to get more out of our exercise and spend less time in the gym, short burst training might be the direction to go.

HEALTH BENEFITS OF SBT

Health is a big motivator for people to exercise: like many of you I wanted a chance to counteract family history, maintain healthy functioning or simply to follow doctor's orders of becoming more fit. There has been research lately on the difference between moderate-intensity long duration training and high-intensity intermittent activity on Relationships of heart disease risk factors to exercise quantity and intensity. Studies showed that exercise intensity had a "13.3 times greater effect on systolic blood pressure, a 2.8 times greater effect on diastolic blood pressure and a 4.7 times greater effect on waist circumference in men than did exercise duration."

MONTH 3 GOALS

o   Training and nutrition are both keys
o   Aim to consume 1.5 gallon of water a day
o   Shoot for consistent intensity each set
o   Weights 4 times weekly
o   Rest 30 seconds between sets
o   1-2 days of recovery cardio if needed (slow and steady for rejuvenation purposes)
o   Learn to enjoy your new body

WORKOUT LOG				
RESISTANCE TRAINING WORKOUT 1/ MONTH 3				
Exercise	SETS 4-6	WEIGHT	TIME 60 SEC	WEEK
Dumbbell Squat to Overhead Press				
Dumbbell High Pull				
Bodyweight Jump Squat				
Push Ups with Hands on Stability Ball				
Plank with 2 Points Contact				
Any Cardio x 3 minutes				

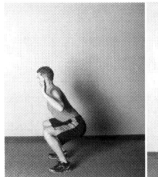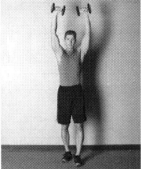

Dumbbell Squat to Overhead Press

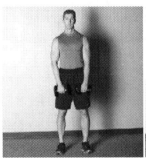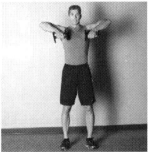

Dumbbell High Pull

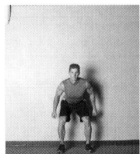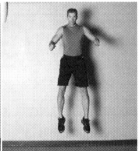

Bodyweight Jump Squat

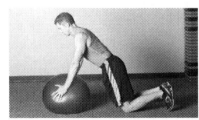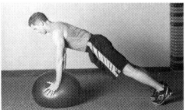

Push-ups with Hands on Stability Ball

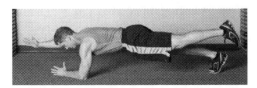

Plank with 2 Contact Points

Dumbbell Squat to Overhead Press:

Start with a pair of dumbbells at shoulder level hands facing in. Lower your body by bending knees into a squatting position while maintaining dumbbells in same position. As you come back up to starting position push hands upward and overhead by extending arms overhead. Lower dumbbells back to starting position and repeat. ***Image shows entry level option and advanced option.**

Dumbbell High Pull:

Start in a standing position holding the dumbbells in front of you. Pulling with you arms, bring the dumbbells to shoulder height. Lower the dumbbells and return to the starting position. Elbows should remain higher than hands throughout movement.

Body Weight Jump Squat:

Start in a deep squat position with arms extended in front of you. From this position, explosively jump up as high as you can and reach for the ceiling with your hands as you jump, land softly on the balls of your feet. If you feel strong hold dumbbells in your hands or a medicine ball.

Push-ups with Hands on Stability Ball:

Get in pushup position with your hands just out from the center of a stability ball. Assume a 2 o'clock and 10 o'clock hand position on the ball. Bend your elbows, lowering body toward the ball. When your chest comes within an inch or two of the ball, press back up. That's one rep.

Plank w/ 2 Points of Contact:

Start by lying face down on the ground. Place your elbows and forearms underneath your chest. Prop yourself up to form a bridge using your toes and forearms. Maintain a flat back and do not allow your hips to sag towards the ground. From this starting position you should extend opposite foot and hand as far out as you can while maintaining a straight body. Your goal is to extend both away from the body instead of trying to lift it higher. This will help keep body in perfect alignment. Feel free to alternate between sides.

WORKOUT LOG				
RESISTANCE TRAINING WORKOUT 2/ MONTH 3				
Exercise	SETS 4-6	WEIGHT	TIME 60 SEC	WEEK
Standing Cable Row				
Hyperextension on Stability Ball				
Medicine Ball Sitting Rotation				
Dumbbell Standing Shrug				
Ab Wheel Roll Out				
Any Cardio x3 minutes				

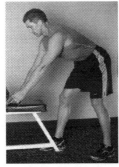
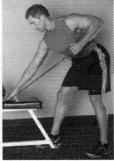

Standing Cable Low Row

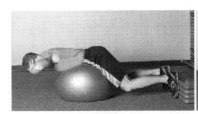

Hyperextension on Stability Ball

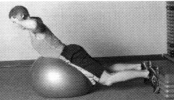

Medicine Ball Sitting Rotation

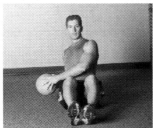
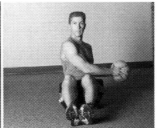

Dumbbell Standing Shrug

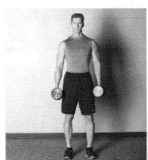
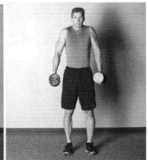

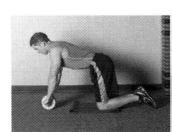
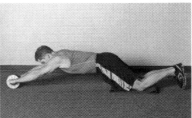

Ab Wheel Roll Out

Standing Cable Low Row:

Stand to side of rotating pulley at medium to low height. Place hand shoulder height or slightly lower on support bar with arm straight. Place foot nearest supporting arm forward with knee slightly bent and opposite foot back. Grasp cable stirrup with one hand allowing shoulder to be pulled forward under weight on cable. Pull cable attachment to side of torso while pulling shoulder back, arching spine, and pushing chest forward. Return until arm is extended and shoulder is pulled forward. Repeat and continue with opposite arm.

Hyperextension on Stability Ball:

Lie prone (on stomach) on ball with knees bent slightly. Feet initially should be propped against an object that will not move (wall, door or weighted box). Position toes on floor for balance. Initiate movement by contracting lower back muscles and posterior leg muscles. Raise torso off of ball by hyper extending spine. Return torso to ball and repeat.

Medicine Ball Rotation in Seated Position:

Sit on butt with knees slightly bent and heels on floor. Tighten abdomen and bounce medicine ball on outside of right knee. Catch the ball and rotate to the left side and repeat.

Dumbbell Standing Shrug:

Standing, grasp dumbbell with hands at sides and raise shoulders as high as you can and then lower to full extension. **TIPS AND TECHNIQUES:** Droop the shoulders down as far as possible and then raise them as high as possible (as though you really, really don't care). The traps are pretty strong so you'll need to pile on the weights.

Ab Wheel Roll Out:

Begin by kneeling on the floor, and hold both sides of the wheel. Use a pad for your knees or kneel on a mat for comfort. Roll the wheel forward, and lower your body as far as you can without arching your back. Then, use you abs to pull yourself back to the starting position. Only go as far as you can control. This is considered advanced, so start off in a small range of movement adding distance after you master the shorter ranges.

Chapter 7: DYNAMIC WARM UP AND SLOW DOWN STRETCHES

It's important to remember that warming up before and slowing down after your workouts are going to be a driving force in preventing new injuries and helping to overcome chronic injuries. I mentioned earlier that warming up and stretching in general are the most under-rated areas in fitness now because most of us who do currently exercise would rather do another set of curls instead of taking 5 minutes to prepare for the curl and another 5 minutes to recover from the curl. It's another case of I want it now and this component of my new life is too slow in the process.

Try focusing instead on taking 5 minutes before and after to get your mind clear so that your exercise experience will be positive and productive. Hard workouts are going to require moments of recovery and reflection. This 5 minutes we are talking about will help clear the clutter that we carry around and free the mind as well as prepare the body for the stresses of the workout and from the day.

The warm up should be used before each workout whether it is resistance training or cardio. The slow down stretches should be performed after every resistance and cardio session. Keep this component alive in your program and you will reap unbelievable rewards in the end. These are just a few warm up and slow down stretches just like the exercises in each workout. Start small and develop your bag of tricks as you progress.

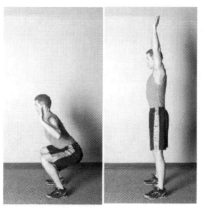

Bodyweight Squat

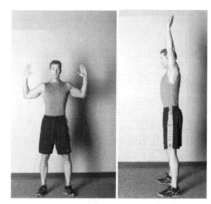

Stick Ups

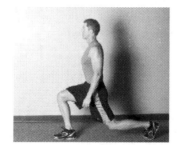

Step Lunge

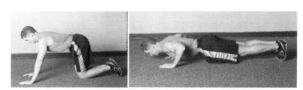

Push Ups

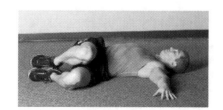

Supine Lower Body Rotation

Warm Ups
Perform 10 reps of each
Bodyweight Squat
Stick Ups
Step Lunge
Push Ups
Supine Lower Body Rotation

WARM-UP CIRCUIT

Complete this warm-up circuit two times, resting 30 seconds between circuits.

Squat(10 reps)

Hold your hands overhead or in front with your feet greater than shoulder-width apart, pushing your hips backward, squat as deep as possible. Push back to the starting position.

Stick-up (10 reps)

Stand with your back against a wall, feet 6 inches away from the wall. Stick your hands up overhead. Keeping your shoulders, elbows, and wrists in contact with the wall, slide your arms down the wall and tuck your elbows into your sides. Return to the starting position.

Pushup (10 reps)

Assume the classic pushup position: legs straight, hands beneath your shoulders. Now brace your abs, keeping your body rigid, lower yourself until your chest touches the floor. Then push back up until your arms are extended. If you are not strong enough to do traditional pushup then simply do them from your knees. ***Image shows entry level option and advanced option.**

Step Lunge (5 reps per leg)

From a standing position, take a large step forward with one leg. When your front thigh is parallel to the floor and your back knee is off the floor, hold for 1 second. Then return to the starting position and repeat with your other leg.

Supine Lower Body Rotation (10 reps per side)

Lie on your back with knees bent and feet close to your butt. Arms are straight to the side like you are making a "t." Keeping knees and feet together simply rotate to the left and back to the right.

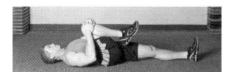

Knee to Chest

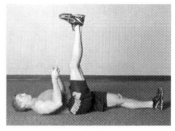

Hamstring

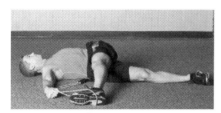

Rotation

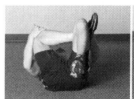

½ Pretzel

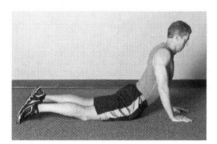

Prone Extension

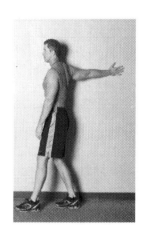

Chest/Biceps

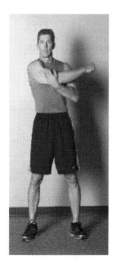

Upper Back Shoulders

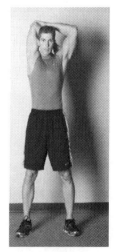

Triceps

Stretches
Hold Each for 10-15 seconds
Knee to Chest
Hamstring
Rotation
1/2 Pretzel
Prone Extension
Chest/Biceps
Upper Back Shoulders
Triceps

Stretches

Perform each stretch 1-2 times every time you workout.

Knee to Chest: (hold 30 seconds each knee)

Lie on your back while grabbing behind your knee gently pull knee towards chest.

Hamstring: (hold 30 seconds each leg)

Lie on back and place towel or band around foot of leg being stretched. Gently pull leg back until stretch / pull is felt behind leg. To enhance stretch make a muscle in upper thigh, this will cause leg to straighten more.

Rotation: (hold 30 seconds each leg)

From hamstring stretch simply put both ends of towel in opposite hand of leg being stretched and slowly pull leg and foot across body trying to rest on floor. Once reaching the floor simply make a muscle in upper thigh again and stretch will be enhanced.

½ Pretzel: (hold 30 seconds each leg)

On back simply cross right foot over left thigh; using left hand pull down softly on right ankle. This will cause stretch in right glute area. Simply pull back on your left knee and bring it towards the chest which will enhance the stretch further.

Prone Extension: (do 10 reps)

Lie on stomach and put hands under body in starting push up position. Instead of picking up lower body off floor push thru hands and upper body will lift up. Try and sag at waist level and stretch will be felt in abdomen area. Be cautious not to over push into hands. See what limitations in abdomen and lower back are first.

Chest / Biceps: (hold 30 seconds each side)

Stand and grab any object that will not move at chest height. Simply apply pressure into palm of hand and rotate upper / lower body away from hand. Stretch will be obvious.

Upper Back and Shoulders: (hold each for 30 seconds)

Take one hand and place it above opposite elbow. Simply pull that arm across body and pressure will be felt on outside of shoulder.

Triceps: (hold for 30 seconds)

Take hand and drop behind head while keeping chin facing forward. Take opposite hand and pull elbow towards the head or midline of the body. Pressure will be felt in shoulder slightly and behind arm.

Chapter 8: TWO NEW LETTERS TO ADD TO YOUR NUTRITIONAL ARSENAL

F and R are the first two letters in the words "fresh or frozen" and this is the way you need to prepare for your weekly shopping. Now-a-days you can walk into any grocery store and buy unbelievable produce that is either fresh or frozen without all of the additives and preservatives and most of all sodium. The frozen food stays fresh as long as you keep the bags sealed and the fresh food speaks for itself. If you are buying fresh meat, fish or poultry then you already know the length of time you can store these foods before they go bad. You can buy local and it helps out the economy in your city as well as fortifying your body with food that it needs to live longer and healthier.

As with weight training, there are nutrition principles that we need to incorporate into each meal of every day.

PRINCIPLE #1: IT'S A LIFESTYLE

For most Americans, it's all about making your health a priority. Most of you reading this book are in need of making changes to your dietary habits to improve the odds that you will live longer. We take things for granted in this country and food is another item that should be added to the list. (What?) You are hard pressed to go to a busy intersection in an average size city and not find that corner overflowing with fast food eateries. What we are going to do is give you insight so that when you are forced into situations that could be labeled a "questionable dietary decision," you stay the course based on the information you have obtained by reading this section of the KISS method.

There is so much information out there that this nutrition topic is probably more confusing than we find with the weight training in earlier chapters. It is no wonder that most Americans and the majority of the kids out there under 15 years of age are labeled fat by academic standards. There are few foods that have taken a beating like the potato. The chart below shows the calories, calories from fat, total fat, sodium, potassium, total carbohydrates, dietary fiber and protein content for a 5.2 ounce potato. For you math whizzes out there that's almost a ½ pound potato.

Serving size = 148 grams or 5.2 ounces	Russet Norkotah	Russet Burbank	Red	Yellow	White
Calories	110	110	100	120	110
Calories from Fat	0	0	0	0	0
Total Fat	0	0	0	0	0
Sodium	10 mg	15 mg	0 mg	0 mg	0 mg
Potassium	680 mg	640 mg	710 mg	810 mg	700 mg
Total Carbohydrates	22 g	23 g	23 g	26 g	25 g
Dietary Fiber	3 g	2 g	2 g	2 g	2 g
Protein	4 g	4 g	3 g	3 g	3 g

There is no fat or sodium (except for the russet variety). So how could something so healthy, get so much bad publicity and be one of the foods that is listed in books like Atkins, Sugar Busters, etc., as a food that you should stay away from? What happens is that we load up this nutrient source with butter, bacon and cheese and then turn it into a heart attack waiting to happen. A few years ago I started adding low fat cottage cheese instead of butter, sour cream or regular cheese to improve the nutritional make up of my potato. Fat levels were kept in check and very little sodium was added to this otherwise healthy partner in the race to live longer.

There are many other foods that have been put into the same category as the potato so my suggestion is: before you take a food away that offers high quality nutrition, simply look at how you or the restaurants you frequent prepares the food.

So here are a few options to look at when eating out.

- There must be a vegetable portion to each meal that you eat and it cannot be fried or sautéed.
- Must have a lean protein portion (chicken, beef, pork or fish)
- Oils and sauces should be on the side
- Cooked light or oil free
- Order off the menu and not get specials (most will have fancy sauces or hidden calories)

- Decide on the meal before you get to a restaurant so that you do not get caught making bad decision. Instead ask them to fax or email you their menu.
- Goal is to keep calories to 500 or less

PRINCIPLE # 2: CHOOSE HIGH QUALITY FOODS

There are different categories of food to discuss. Carbohydrates can be broken down into vegetables, fruit and starchy options like bread or pasta. Protein and fat sources come from fish, meat, poultry, pork, nuts, eggs and some vegetables like the avocado. Some of the foods fall into multiple categories like the avocado. It is a great source of good fats and protein and carbohydrate while still being a vegetable.

A major consideration is the portion size of some foods you eat. Foods that are high in fat (even if it is a good fat like those from cold water fish, avocado and nuts) are going to be higher in calories per gram of weight than an equal weight of broccoli or cabbage. The average fat gram has 9 calories where the average protein and carbohydrate gram have only 4 calories. So, for those of you trying to lose weight this should be factored in since fat has twice the calories as carbohydrates and lean protein sources. Listed below will be guidelines to follow with each category so that you can make informed choices.

CARBOHYDRATES FROM VEGETABLE GUIDELINES
- Fresh or frozen instead of canned
- The exceptions are tomatoes, artichokes, bell peppers and hearts of palm

CARBOHYDRATES FROM FRUIT GUIDLINES
- Fresh or frozen instead of canned unless frozen way is saucy

CARBOYDRATES FROM STARCHES GUIDELINES
- Fiber : Carbohydrate ratio should be 1 or more grams fiber to 10 grams of carbohydrates
- Cannot say enriched on ingredients list
- Fiber exceptions include rice and pasta (remember it is the combination of sauces or preparation that causes these foods to become unhealthy)

PROTEIN GUIDELINES
- Low fat except for eggs and fish

In order to optimize your food you should also drink water with every meal, eat a fruit and / or a vegetable with each meal, eat at least 3 protein servings every day and eat healthy fats daily. Remember that you are helping with this process of incorporating a new healthier lifestyle in order to achieve longer living potential. So, do the homework and check to see if the foods you love now fall into the healthy or unhealthy category and if so, what can you do to help in the salvaging process with the unhealthy foods.

PRINCIPLE #3: EAT IN A HEALTHY MEAL PATTERN

How many times have you heard or read something about eating every 2-4 hours? It's everywhere. Ask yourself this question, "***If it were not important to living healthier and maintaining a healthy weight, would it be available from every media outlet imaginable?***" This principal is the basic foundation to achieving long lasting positive effects in your life journey. By eating more and smaller meals (4-6 meals of 300-500 calories each) you are keeping your body from starving and tearing down the muscle you do have for energy.

As soon as you start to exercise you are going to need more energy to fuel these increasingly more demanding workouts and also aid in the recovery from each workout. You will start to notice that when you pay attention to the healthy foods you do put into your body they are going to make you feel better because they are not enriched with additives like sodium. These healthier foods are going to be nutrient rich but not high in calories. Look at a bag of frozen vegetables (mixed) from Birds Eye that weighs 12 oz. A serving size is 2/3 of a cup and there are 4 servings in the bag. Each serving has 0 fat and 60 calories. So by eating the whole bag you would have taken in 240 calories and 0 fat grams. Pair this with a lean protein source or some nuts and you will have a balanced meal that will not leave you feeling empty or hungry in a couple hours. So the next time you are scheduled to eat you will not have to stuff your face. This is how we can keep calories per meal to 300-500.

My suggestion is to save your meal(s) that have a higher concentration of carbohydrates from starches till after your workout. This will give your muscles the needed fuel to recover from your workouts and keep your mind sharp for the rest of your day or night.

Keeping this section realistic is the most important decision that you have to make. My lifestyle and career put me in an environment that allows me to receive support daily. It might be harder for some of you reading this book to get the support you need or to make sure that every single meal fits into the 3 principles mentioned above because of picky eating habits or children. If you start now trying to make more, better decisions than bad ones then you have already taken the first step to improving your long-term health which is the focus of the book. It's not about being perfect all of the time because life happens!

Chapter 9: SERVING SIZE AND PANTRY MAKEOVER

What does my fridge; freezer and pantry makeover look like?

With the theme of this book being extending your life expectancy I would be remiss if I did not list the types of foods that will help with increasing your odds.

Carbohydrate Source				
Grains	Starchy Vegetables	Beans	Non Starchy Vegetables	Fruits
Quinoa Oatmeal (not the sweetened kind) Brown/wild rice High fiber cereals (Kashi for example) Bran	Potatoes Corn	Black Navy White Garbanzo Red Lentils	Spinach Tomatoes Broccoli Carrots Bell peppers Onions Zucchini Squash Cucumber Cauliflower Romaine lettuce	Apples Oranges (Tangelos, Satsuma, tangerines, etc) Bananas Red grapes Peaches Plums Pineapple Avocado Strawberry Blueberry Blackberry Raspberry All melons

Protein Source			
Meats	Dairy	Supplements	Fats
Extra lean ground beef Lean beef Skinless chicken Turkey Lean pork Deer Buffalo Salmon Tuna Cod Egg whites (use the yolks sparingly)	Yogurt Cottage cheese Milk Cheeses	Creatine Protein Powder Blend	Olive oil Flax seed oil Flaxmeal Avocado Almonds Walnuts Macadamia Cashews Fish oil caps

Here is the crazy part of the nutrition plan. As you look over the food options here, remember that balance is the name of the game. If you do not like certain foods that are listed, take it upon yourself to look for foods that would be in the same family as the ones listed above and try them. Remember that it comes down to you fueling your body with healthier foods that will ultimately make you fit, healthy and happy. There are countless resources on the web and all you have to do is look for it in a search engine. But be careful, some might include false info, so make sure you are using a reliable source. If you have allergies to certain foods then I can almost guarantee there is a similar food available that will not cause you to have a reaction. If you are not a breakfast person have another lunch or dinner meal, just don't skip meals altogether.

SERVING SIZES

Most people know about the Food Guide Pyramid. They also know why we need to eat food from each of the five groups each day. Many also know the number of servings from each group that are needed each day, but many do not know what a serving is.

You may be eating good foods each day, but still are not as healthy as you could be because of the **amount** of food you eat. The amount of food you eat can be as important to your good health as what you eat.

SERVINGS AND SIZES NEEDED

Here is a review of the number of servings needed each day from each of the food groups and some ways to picture a serving size using everyday objects. Using these examples may help you see you are eating more servings from the Food Guide Pyramid than you think.

Bread, Cereal, Rice, and Pasta (6 to 11 servings)	
A serving is:	Picture:
1 slice of bread	audio cassette tape
1/2 cup of cooked cereal, rice, or pasta	tennis ball or ice cream scoop

Vegetables (3 to 5 servings)	
A serving is:	Picture:
3/4 cup tomato juice	small Styrofoam cup
1 cup salad greens	baseball
1/2 cup cooked broccoli	scoop of ice cream
1/2 cup cooked or chopped raw vegetables	6 asparagus spears; 7 or 8 baby carrots or carrot sticks or 1 ear of corn on the cob

Fruits (2 to 4 servings)	
A serving is:	Picture:
1/2 cup of grapes (15 grapes)	size of a light bulb
1 medium size fruit (apple, banana, orange,…)	tennis ball

Meat, Poultry, Fish, Dry Beans, Eggs and Nuts (2 to 3 servings)	
A serving is:	Picture:
1 tablespoon peanut butter	ping pong ball
3 ounces cooked meat, fish, poultry	deck of cards or a cassette tape
3 ounces cooked chicken	chicken leg and thigh or breast

Milk, Yogurt, and Cheese (2 to 3 servings)	
A serving is:	Picture:
1 1/2 ounces cheese	9 volt battery or 3 dominoes
1 ounce of cheese	pair of dice
1 cup of ice cream	baseball

Fats, Oil, and Sweets (use sparingly)	
A serving is:	Picture:
1 teaspoon butter, margarine	stamp or the thickness of a pencil
2 tablespoons salad dressing	ping pong ball

When preparing to take photos for this book I weighed 204 lbs. and had a body fat percentage around 11. I decided that in order to add validity to the book I wanted to try out the different dietary suggestions that I was asking you to follow and track my progress over a 6-week period. Keep in mind that I already was a healthy eater and outside of the 1-2 glasses of "medicinal" wine most nights, I only changed a few things. These changes are listed below.

- I cut out all processed or refined foods (bread, etc.) after my lunch meal.
- No products coming out of a can except for tomatoes.
- No more than 3 protein drinks a week because I wanted to eat more real food.
- Drinking on date night only. During date night there were no limits. I found that less alcohol was consumed on that special night than I would have before.

- I watched the amount of salt in the foods I ate and added no extra salt to the food I prepared. Instead I added fresh spices and herbs.
- I added a 3 egg omelet with 1 fork full of fat free cottage cheese every night except date night. I did not wake up hungry the next morning and therefore did not overeat at breakfast.

The end result staggered me. Over the course of the 6-weeks I dropped an amazing 20 lbs. Body fat dropped to single digits and I felt great. The amazing thing is that I was not hungry except for the last 3 days before the photo shoot which was due to me cutting everything out except for asparagus, boiled chicken (not a misprint) and eggs. This was to get the water out from between the muscles. Here is where trying to be perfect is not always realistic. Original photo shoot was to take place on Friday. Thursday morning I get the phone call that my photographer had to cancel and move the photo shoot to the following Tuesday which meant trying to find the balance between taking in enough calories to keep my muscle lean and not overeating or under eating and appearing soft. As most of you can relate to, the thought of boiled chicken and asparagus as your only food sources for 2-3 days causes you to shake with disgust. For most of us one meal of those 2 would be enough. My point here is that life happens, and things rarely go the way we originally plan and it is important to roll with the information and do the best you can.

The pictures came out great and working with my photographer was an incredible experience. I missed my perfect book look by a day but the point here is that my overall appearance and health improved drastically. The best part was that I stuck to a plan because of a personal goal I set. Exercise and eating healthy have always been priorities of mine since turning 18. Having a specific goal was key to my ultimate success!

Chapter 10: VISITING AN OLD FRIEND

So, to revisit an old friend, is it better to workout longer or shorter? Once again, it's a combination of both. When preparing for my boards and different certifications I often enjoyed getting on the elliptical for an hour and reviewing my material from the day. It was a way for me to reconnect in detail with information covered earlier and at the same time get in more exercise when time was available to do so. Keep in mind that I am part of the 10 percent of the population that truly loves to exercise. Short Burst Training garners better, quicker results if time is an issue. But we are talking about bringing balance to your life and finding enjoyment in this journey of exercise. So, if you find yourself needing slower paced activity on occasion then by all means do so.

KISS is set up to take you thru multiple types of training so that your body has time to adjust to the different levels or demands on your energy system(s). This is why your initial visit to your primary care physician is so important. He or she can release you to start exercising without you having to be concerned about overtraining. So, take the time and go get the initial evaluation.

Good luck, train hard and by all means live a healthier, longer life!

Chapter 11: TESTIMONIALS

"How I Did It"

Carole Lamar

Last year I lost 18 pounds. That's a respectable amount of weight but more so for me as on a good day I'm almost 5'2", so it made a big difference in my appearance. Now in my 50's, I had been carrying around the 10 or so extra pounds that plague so many people. I had been working with my trainer, Carey Long, for four years mainly focusing on weight training to combat the prospect of osteoporosis. Cardio wasn't my thing. I hated it but spent a little time on the elliptical machine on an inconsistent basis.

The turning point for me was my husband's upcoming 60th birthday, a milestone birthday that was to be celebrated with family and friends on a trip that would require wearing a swimsuit...a lot. I looked at myself and wasn't pleased with what I saw. I had convinced myself that I was past the point of losing weight and really getting in shape. Carey and I discussed this at length and he convinced me that I could, indeed, accomplish this if I made some changes and stayed the course. It would require making changes in my diet and moving more. The switch in my head turned on and I knew I was committed to achieving my goal. The birthday trip was in June. I began my mission in March.

The first thing I decided to do was cut out any alcohol for a least one month. With my mind made up, this wasn't hard to do. I started keeping a food diary, writing down everything that went into my mouth. Chicken became my new best friend. Salads without dressing, avocadoes, blueberries (also good food for your brain), yogurt, sushi and vegetables became the staples of my diet. These were already some of my favorite foods. Carbohydrates were limited. As I love sugar, I allowed myself one Skinny Cow ice cream sandwich a day.

I continued the weight training with Carey 3 times a week but started doing more cardio than I ever had before. The elliptical machine was easy on my knees, so I tried to spend 30 minutes on it four days a week, pushing it as hard as I could. One week went by. Nothing. I conveyed my disappointment to Carey and he assured me that my body was fighting losing the weight it was used to carrying around and, also, it was resisting resetting my metabolism. Week two went by. I continued to work hard. I was still being consistent with my diet and exercise. Nothing. Not an ounce had I lost. My frustration and disappointment was increasing to the point where I was considering quitting. Maybe I had been right. I was beyond the point of losing weight and being fit. Week three. I started losing weight! It was starting to happen. You can't imagine my excitement and recommitment to continue. Then something else entered my regime. Carey taught a spin class twice a week and had been encouraging me to try it. It looked pretty scary to me. I had seen the people coming out of that spin room dripping with sweat and it didn't look like a whole lot of fun. But, being curious about it, I decided to give it a try. I thought I was going to die. My heart was going to burst, my legs were barely making it after the "warm up" but I forced myself through 40 of the longest minutes of my life.

For some reason, I went back 2 days later. It was still difficult but not as bad as the first time. Then I bought a heart rate monitor and saw the amount of calories that were being burned by spinning. It was amazing. I was hooked.

By the time of the trip in June, I had lost 15 pounds and my body was toned like it had never been before. I had "good arms" for the very first time in my life. Until now, I had always worn long sleeves because I hated my fat arms, now everything I wore was sleeveless. A friend I hadn't seen in months called me one day to ask how she could get her arms to look like mine. She called them Madonna arms. Wow. Me?

Over a year and a half have gone by and I still watch what I eat, still train with Carey 3 times a week and I still spin. And, I've kept the weight off. If I gain 2 or 3 pounds, I know what I need to do to get it off. It's been a good ride.

Diane Kirtland

When I turned 50 a few years back girlfriends took me to Cozumel to celebrate. I had been participating in Pilate's classes 3 times weekly for almost 6 years and thought my physical appearance was maxed out and I looked good. That was until I saw pictures from the trip a few weeks later. My arms had more cellulite than I ever expected. This was totally unacceptable and I contacted Carey at the urging of a friend that had been training with him as well. Within a few months my arms looked great and the same girlfriends that arranged the Cozumel trip were shocked with the arm definition in such a short time. We focused our efforts on getting me stronger which was the beginning of me building toned arms (not bulging mind you). This same effort of building my strength was forwarded to my legs, shoulders, core and back and a leaner me started to surface. How many 50 plus females do you know who can leg press 5-45 pound plates on each side for sets of 12-15 reps? I have never at any point looked like a body builder. Instead, I am proud to wear strapless dresses and have my jeans fit. I had always been afraid of lifting heavier weights because of the "bulking process" that my muscles would go thru and the risk of injury associated. I understand now that by lifting properly injury is reduced significantly and that I am not physically able to have manly muscles.

I am proud of how far my physical and mental well-being has come and I discuss this with friends the need to add resistance movements to build muscle. Some of these same girlfriends started exercising with Carey with similar results.

EXERCISE TERMINOLOGY
Simple meanings for fitness terminology!

Aerobic Exercise
Exercise fitness low-intensity, sustained activity that relies on oxygen for energy. Aerobic activity builds endurance, burns fat and conditions the cardiovascular system.

Anaerobic
High-intensity exercise that burns glycogen for energy, instead of oxygen. Anaerobic exercise creates a temporary oxygen debt by consuming more oxygen than the body can supply. An example of anaerobic exercise includes weight lifting.

Circuit Weight Training
An exercise fitness routine which combines light to moderate-intensity weight training with aerobic training. The object is to move from station to station with little rest between exercises, until the entire circuit has been completed.

Flexibility
The ability of a bone joint or muscle to stretch.

Intensity
The amount of force - or energy - you expend during a workout.

Maximum Heart Rate
The **fastest rate** at which your heart should beat during exercise. To find your maximum rate, subtract your age from 220 for men and 226 for women.

Progressive Overload
The amount of resistance against which a muscle is required to work that exceeds the weight which it normally handles.

Progression
To systematically increase the stress a muscle endures during an exercise fitness routine. Progression is achieved in one of three ways: by increasing the weight in an exercise, by increasing the number of repetitions performed in one set, by increasing the number of sets, or by decreasing the rest interval between sets.

Prone

Movement that occurs while being on your stomach.

Reps / Repetition

When an exercise has progressed through one complete range of motion and back to the beginning, one repetition has been completed, i.e., such as lifting a weight up and down once.

Resistance

The actual weight against which a muscle is working.

Set

This is a series of repetitions done without rest, i.e., such as 10 reps = 1 set.

Stretching

Exercise which increases the ease and degree to which a muscle or joint can turn, bend or reach.

Supine

Movement that occurs while on your back.

GOOD LUCK AND TRAIN HARD!

Visit my website at kissfitness.net to contact me directly.

SPECIAL THANKS!

I need to give a special thanks to my co-workers and training peers. The constant sharing of information and ideas has helped with providing material for this book. Dr. Alvin Granowsky for encouraging me to share my passion with you in the form of a workbook titled **KISS FITNESS**. Katie Pryor for helping me edit the information contained in **KISS FITNESS**. And, my partner Joe for being there with encouragement and a smile when I stumbled during the writing of this project.